DOUGLAS MARK OLSEN JR DMD

Dentistry With Kids

A Parent's Guide To Making Every Dental Visit a Success

I would like to dedicate this work to my children, Audrey and Maverick. You inspire me in all I do and were the major inspiration to write this book to help other parents and children.

Contents

1

Introduction

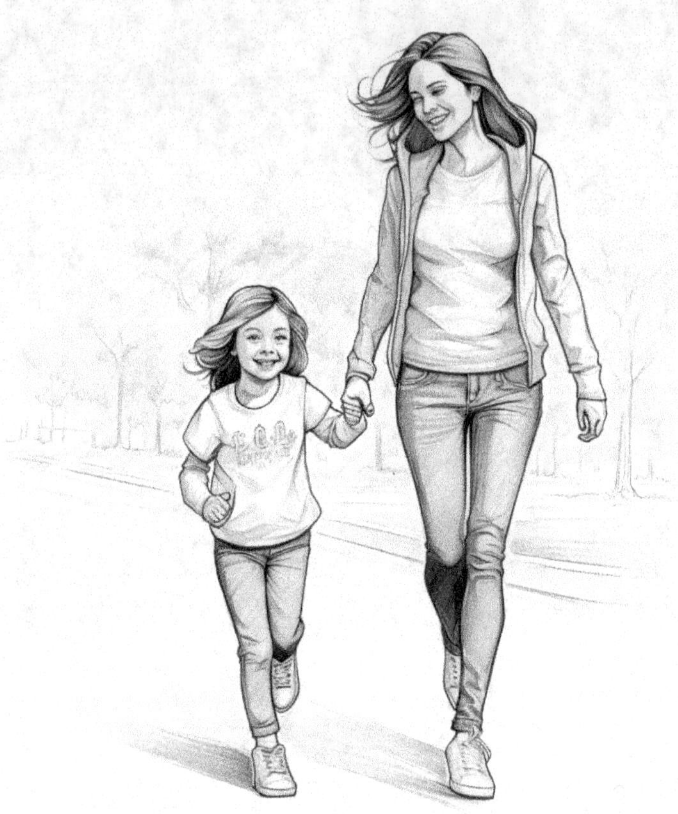

Welcome to "Dentistry With Kids: A Parent's Guide to Making Every Dental Visit a Success," a practical and heartfelt guide crafted to transform your child's dental visits. Even though I'm a dentist, I am first and foremost a parent. I understand the unique challenges and anxieties that come with navigating dental care for your children. Whether you've faced your own dental fears or have sat through a challenging appointment with your little one, this book is your ally and guide.

After years of working in a community health center setting and seeing countless children (and adults as well) struggle with dental anxiety I have continued to wonder what more I could do to help. For a while now I have had the thought that if parents could approach dental treatment the right way with their children it would greatly reduce the overall struggle so many have with dental care.

Dental appointments can be a source of significant stress for both parents and children. But with the right preparation and mindset, these visits can become a positive, even enjoyable, experience. That's not just hopeful thinking; it's entirely possible, and I'm here to show you how.

This material for this book comes from the culmination of personal experiences, professional insights, and real-life success. It's designed to equip you with the tools and knowledge to prepare your child for dental appointments, support them during the process, and ensure a positive aftermath. Each chapter is packed with actionable advice, easy-to-implement strategies, and empathetic understanding.

From the first chapter, 'Before the Appointment: Preparing for Success,' we'll explore how to lay a solid foundation for a positive dental experience. This includes understanding your child's fears, communicating effectively about the dentist, and everything you need to set your child up for success.

In 'During the Appointment,' we dive into practical tips for the day of the visit. You'll learn how to support your child, collaborate with the dental team, and use techniques to reduce anxiety and fear.

The journey doesn't end there. 'After the Appointment' covers post-visit care, how to debrief with your child, and fostering a positive ongoing relationship with dental health.

"Dentistry With Kids" isn't just a book; it's a roadmap to transforming dental visits into successful, stress-free experiences. It's about empowering you, the parent, and giving your child the gift of a lifetime: a healthy, happy relationship with dental care!

Before the Appointment, Preparing for Success

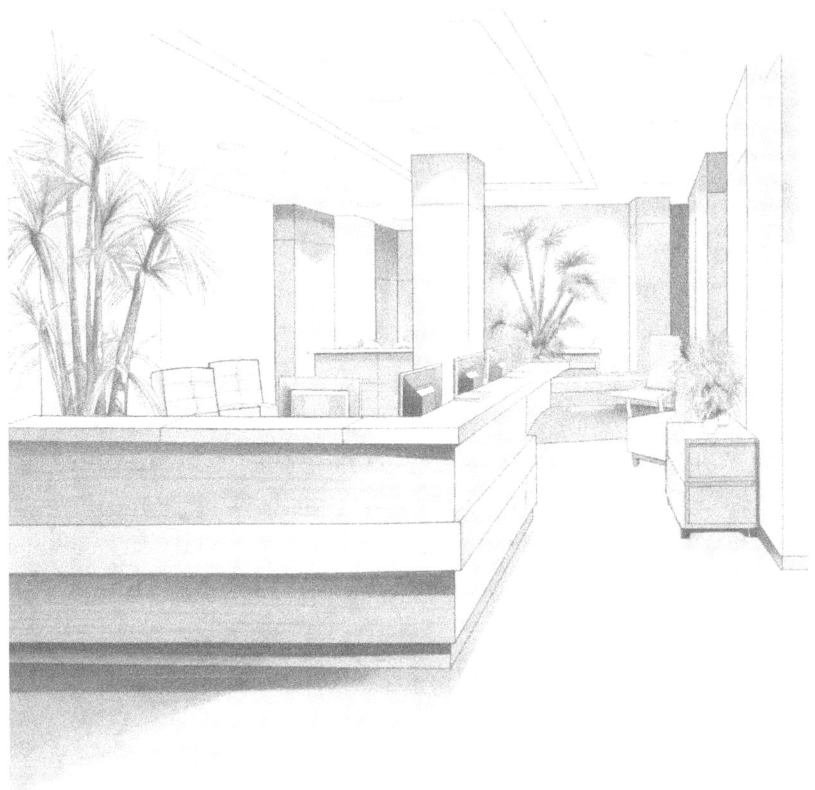

Having a good, positive dental visit with your child begins long before you step into the dentist's office. The groundwork for a successful appointment is laid through thoughtful preparation and a positive mindset. This chapter will be your guide for preparing your child to have a great experience.

Age of First Appointment: Embracing Early Dental Visits

When should your child's dental journey begin? The journey to dental success starts early! The American Academy of Pediatric Dentistry recommends the first dental visit by age one or within six months after the first tooth erupts. This early start may seem surprising, but it's grounded in sound reasoning.

Firstly, early visits are all about prevention. Dental problems can start early, and the sooner a dentist can identify issues, the better. It's not just about checking for cavities; these initial visits allow dentists to examine the development of your child's jaw, assess any potential alignment issues, and guide you on teething and oral hygiene practices.

Secondly, early visits set a precedent. They help in normalizing the experience of going to the dentist. For a child, the dental office can be a place of curiosity rather than fear. Familiarizing your child with the environment, the sounds, and the routine of dental check-ups at a young age can lay the groundwork for stress-free future visits.

Moreover, these visits are educational for parents too. They offer a golden opportunity to learn about proper oral care for your child, dietary advice for healthy teeth, and habits to avoid, like prolonged bottle-feeding. Remember, it's not just about that one tooth; it's about setting up a lifetime of good oral health.

In essence, the age of the first dental appointment is a crucial milestone in your child's health journey. It's an investment in their oral health, an educational opportunity for you, and a chance to cultivate a positive relationship between your child and dental care. So, embrace this early start with enthusiasm and confidence, knowing you're paving the way for your child's lifelong dental wellbeing.

Choosing a Dentist: Finding the Right Match for Your Child

Selecting the right dentist for your child is a decision that goes far beyond convenience and location. It's about finding a professional who can provide not only excellent dental care but also a positive, nurturing experience. Here's why choosing a dentist experienced with children and with whom you feel comfortable is crucial.

Experience with Children is Key

Pediatric dentists specialize in treating children, and their offices are typically designed to be child-friendly, often with playful decor and engaging activities to create a welcoming atmosphere. Their training goes beyond dental care; they understand child psychology and know how to communicate with children in a way that makes them feel safe and at ease. This specialized approach can make a significant difference in how your child perceives dental visits. Many general dentists are great with children and provide dental care to children at the same level as a pediatric dentist. The key is doing your research and making a good educated choice on who you trust with the care of your child.

Comfort Level with the Dentist

Your comfort with the dentist is just as important as your child's. When you trust and feel at ease with the dentist, it naturally translates to a more positive experience for your child. You're more likely to have an open line of communication, discuss concerns freely, and feel confident in the care your child is receiving. This trust is essential, as it allows for effective collaboration in maintaining and improving your child's oral health.

Finding the Right Fit

So, how do you find this perfect match? Start by seeking recommendations from friends, family, or your child's pediatrician. Online reviews and parents' forums can also offer valuable insights. Once you have a few options, consider visiting the dental offices. Observe the environment and how staff interact with children. Is the atmosphere welcoming and kid-friendly? Are the staff patient and accommodating?

Don't hesitate to ask questions. Inquire about the dentist's experience with children, their approach to dealing with anxious or nervous young patients, and their philosophy on dental care for kids. Your goal is to find a dentist who is not only qualified but also aligns with your values and approach to health care.

Choosing the right dentist for your child is a blend of professional expertise and personal rapport. It's about finding a place where your child can build positive associations with dental care, ensuring their oral health journey is off to the best start possible. Take your time, do your research, and trust your instincts – after all, no one knows your child better than you do.

Your Child's Mood: Setting the Stage for a Positive Experience

The mood and overall well-being of your child on the day of the dental appointment can significantly influence how the visit unfolds. Ensuring your child is well-rested, well-fed, and generally in good spirits can be as crucial as the appointment itself. Here's how to set your child up for success.

A Good Night's Sleep

A well-rested child is typically more cooperative and better able to handle new or unfamiliar situations. Ensure your child gets a full night's sleep before the day of the dental visit. A regular bedtime routine, free from overstimulation, can help in achieving this. A rested child will be more alert, less irritable, and better equipped emotionally to handle the dental visit.

Nutrition Matters

Hunger can make anyone cranky, especially a child. Make sure your child has a nutritious meal before the appointment. This not only keeps their energy levels up but also helps in stabilizing their mood. However, avoid sugary foods or drinks as they can lead to a spike in energy levels, potentially making your child more restless or hyperactive during the visit. Opt for meals that are filling and provide sustained energy.

Hydration is Key

Keeping your child well-hydrated is also important. Dehydration can lead to irritability and discomfort, so ensure your child drinks enough water before the visit. However, be mindful of the timing to avoid the need for frequent bathroom breaks during the appointment.

Avoid Overstimulation

Before the appointment, try to keep the environment calm and relaxed. Overstimulation from activities or screen time can lead to restlessness, making it harder for your child to remain calm and seated during the dental visit. Encourage activities that are soothing or gently engaging.

Setting the Emotional Tone

Your child can pick up on your emotions, so it's important to manage your own anxieties and remain calm and positive. If you're relaxed and upbeat about the visit, your child is more likely to mirror those feelings. Keep the conversation about the dentist positive and light, focusing on the benefits of having healthy teeth.

Your child's mood plays a significant role in the success of a dental visit. By ensuring they are well-rested, well-fed, and in a positive state of mind, you're laying the foundation for a smooth and successful dental experience. This proactive approach not only helps in making the visit more pleasant but also reinforces positive associations with dental care for the future.

Being Positive and Encouraging: Fostering Confidence and Courage

The power of your words and attitude in shaping your child's perception of the dentist cannot be overstated. Positive reinforcement and encouraging dialogue play a pivotal role in building your child's confidence and reducing any potential anxiety. Here's how to use positivity and encouragement effectively.

Speak Encouraging Words

Start by talking to your child about the dentist in an upbeat and positive tone. Highlight how the dentist helps keep teeth strong and healthy. Use simple, child-friendly language to explain what they do, focusing on the positive aspects, like how the dentist can make teeth shiny and clean or how they're like superheroes for teeth.

Praise Their Bravery

Children respond well to praise and encouragement. Tell your child how brave and grown-up they are for going to the dentist. Acknowledge that it's okay to feel nervous, but emphasize how proud you are of them for overcoming their fears. This affirmation can boost their self-confidence and make them more receptive to the dental experience.

Create a Positive Narrative

Use storytelling or role-play to create a positive narrative around the dental visit. You could tell a story about a favorite character who had a fun time visiting the dentist or play pretend dentist at home. This not only makes the idea of visiting the dentist more familiar but also fun and engaging.

Avoid Negative Language

Steer clear of any language that suggests pain, discomfort, or fear. Even saying, "It won't hurt" can plant the idea of pain. Instead, focus on the positive aspects and maintain an upbeat tone. Avoid sharing any negative dental experiences you may have had; children can easily pick up on these fears.

Visualize a Positive Experience

Encourage your child to imagine the visit going well. Talk about what they might see and hear, and how good they will feel after the visit. Visualization can be a powerful tool in building a positive mindset.

In essence, being positive and encouraging is about creating an environment of safety, trust, and optimism. Your words and attitude can significantly influence your child's feelings towards dental care. By consistently using positive reinforcement and encouraging language, you're not just preparing them for a successful dental visit; you're helping them develop a resilient and confident approach to new experiences.

Tell Them What to Expect: Demystifying the Dental Visit

Children often fear the unknown, and the dentist's office is no exception. By explaining what will happen during the visit in a clear, child-friendly way, you can help alleviate their anxiety. Here's how to prepare your child by setting clear, positive expectations for their dental appointment.

Describe the Dental Procedures Simply

Start by explaining the basic procedures in simple terms. Tell your child that the dentist will be cleaning their teeth, which helps keep them shiny and healthy. You can compare it to how they clean their toys to keep them looking nice. Mention that the dentist will count and check their teeth, looking for 'sugar bugs' (cavities) and making sure their teeth are strong.

Explain the Importance of Oral Hygiene

Let your child know that the dentist will teach them how to take care of their teeth properly. Explain that this is like learning superpowers to fight against cavity-causing germs. Emphasize how they'll learn to brush like a hero, keeping their smile bright and healthy.

Introduce Them to Dental Instruments

Familiarize your child with some of the tools the dentist might use. For example, you can describe the small mirror as a tool to see all the teeth's nooks and crannies and the explorer as a special tooth counter to make sure all their teeth are there. Keeping the descriptions light and fun can reduce fear of the unknown.

Talk About X-rays in a Fun Way

If X-rays are a part of the visit, explain them as a special camera that can take pictures of their teeth. You can liken it to a superhero gadget that helps the dentist see how their teeth are doing inside their mouth.

Normalize the Experience

Share with your child that everyone, including you, visits the dentist regularly to keep their teeth healthy. You can talk about your own positive experiences or those of their favorite characters or role models. This normalization helps them understand that dental visits are a regular part of life.

Use Positive Reinforcement

Reassure your child that the dentist's job is to help and that they are there to make sure their teeth are in the best shape. Remind them of how brave and grown-up they are for going to the dentist and how proud you are of them for taking care of their teeth.

Telling your child what to expect at the dentist in an age-appropriate and positive way can transform uncertainty into curiosity and fear into bravery. By demystifying the dental visit, you not only prepare them for what's to come but also help build their confidence and trust in dental care, setting the stage for a lifetime of healthy smiles.

Do Not Scare Your Child: Creating a Fear-Free Narrative

One of the most important aspects of preparing your child for a dental visit is ensuring that the narrative around it is free of fear and anxiety. It's crucial to control the flow of information your child receives about dental visits, especially from sources that might instill fear, such as older siblings or even your own past experiences. Here's how to maintain a positive atmosphere.

Avoid Sharing Negative Stories

Children are impressionable, and they can easily absorb the fears and anxieties of those around them. Be mindful of the conversations you have about dental visits in front of your child. Avoid discussing any negative experiences you or others may have had. Even if you have had less than pleasant experiences, focus on the positive aspects of dental care and its importance for health.

Monitor Conversations with Siblings

Older siblings can unintentionally scare younger children with tales of dental visits. It's important to talk to any older children in the family and explain the importance of keeping dental discussions positive. Encourage them to share encouraging stories or support their younger sibling's dental journey with positive reinforcement.

Reframe Scary Concepts

If your child has already heard something frightening about the dentist, take the time to reframe these ideas. For instance, if they've heard about 'drills' or 'needles,' explain that dentists have special tools to gently take care of teeth, and they always make sure the child is comfortable and safe.

Create a Safe Space for Questions

Encourage your child to ask questions about the dentist and answer them honestly yet positively. If you don't know the answer, it's okay to say so and suggest finding out together. This open dialogue can alleviate fears stemming from misinformation or imagination.

Reinforce Positive Messages

Continually reinforce the idea that the dentist is a friend who helps keep their teeth strong and healthy. Highlight the positive outcomes of dental visits, like a bright smile and healthy teeth. Use positive language and imagery when discussing dental topics.

Lead by Example

Children often mirror the attitudes and behaviors of their parents. Show a calm and positive demeanor when discussing or going to the dentist. If possible, let your child see you having a positive dental experience. This modeling can be very powerful in shaping their perceptions.

Ensuring that the narrative around dental visits is free of fear involves careful management of the information your child receives and how it is presented. By maintaining a positive dialogue, encouraging open communication, and leading by example, you can create a supportive and reassuring environment that helps dispel any fears associated with dental visits. This approach not only prepares them for a successful dental experience but also contributes to their overall emotional well-being.

3

During the Appointment

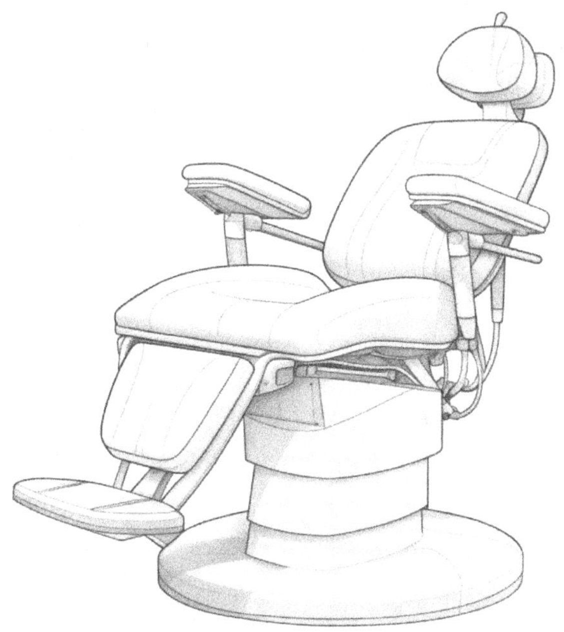

The day of the dental appointment has arrived, and as a parent, your role is pivotal in ensuring the visit goes smoothly. This chapter is dedicated to guiding you on how you can be most helpful during the appointment, creating an atmosphere of calm and support for your child.

Be Early: Setting a Calm and Prepared Tone

Arriving early for your child's dental appointment is a small step that can have a big impact on the overall experience. Being punctual is not just about being respectful of the dentist's schedule; it's about creating a calm, unrushed atmosphere for both you and your child. Here's why arriving early is beneficial.

Time to Fill Out Paperwork

Dental appointments often require paperwork, especially if it's your child's first visit or if there are updates to your insurance or medical history. Arriving early gives you ample time to fill out these forms without feeling hurried. This calm start is crucial because children are incredibly perceptive and can easily pick up on your stress or anxiety.

Reducing Stress for Both Parent and Child

When you're not rushed, you're more likely to remain calm and relaxed. This sense of tranquility is infectious; your child will likely feel more at ease if they sense that you're composed and unhurried. A relaxed start can set a positive tone for the rest of the visit.

Time for Acclimatization

Arriving with time to spare allows your child to gradually acclimate to the dental office environment. They can observe other children having positive interactions with the staff, explore the waiting area, or engage with any toys or books available. This period of acclimatization can significantly reduce any initial apprehension or anxiety your child might feel.

Opportunity for Last-Minute Reassurance

This extra time also provides an opportunity for you to offer last-minute reassurance and answer any questions your child might have. You can calmly discuss what will happen during the appointment, reinforce that the dentist is there to help, and remind them of how brave they are.

Building a Routine

Consistently arriving early can help establish a routine, making dental visits a predictable and familiar experience for your child. Over time, this can contribute to reducing dental anxiety and building positive associations with dental care.

Being early for a dental appointment is more than just a matter of punctuality. It's about ensuring you and your child are in the best possible frame of mind for the visit. By arriving early, filling out paperwork in a relaxed manner, and taking the time to acclimate and reassure your child, you are setting the stage for a successful and stress-free dental experience.

Be Kind and Encouraging: Maintaining a Supportive Atmosphere

During your child's dental appointment, your demeanor plays a crucial role in shaping their experience. Being kind and encouraging, and maintaining a composed attitude even in moments of potential stress, can greatly influence how your child perceives and reacts to the visit. Here's how to be the supportive anchor your child needs.

Maintain a Positive Demeanor

Throughout the appointment, it's important to keep your interactions with your child, the dental staff, and the dentist as positive and gentle as possible. Offer your child smiles, words of encouragement, and reassurance. Praise their bravery and cooperation, and remind them of how proud you are. This positive reinforcement can help ease any nerves they may have.

Avoid Showing Frustration

It's natural to feel anxious or concerned during your child's dental visit, especially if they become upset or if the appointment doesn't go as planned. However, try to manage these feelings without showing frustration. Children are adept at picking up on emotional cues, and your anxiety or irritation could inadvertently heighten their own.

Ask Questions Calmly

If you have questions or concerns, by all means, ask them, but do so in a non-confrontational and calm manner. Whether it's a query about a dental procedure, treatment plan, or something you observe during the appointment, approach the conversation with a desire to understand, rather than to challenge. Clear, respectful communication can lead to more informative and constructive discussions.

Collaborate with the Dental Staff

View the dentist and their team as your allies in ensuring the best care for your child. Work with them, offering any necessary information about your child's health or behavior that might be helpful. If your child is particularly anxious or has special needs, share this with the dentist beforehand so they can prepare accordingly.

Lead by Example

Demonstrate to your child how to interact respectfully and kindly with the dental staff. Showing respect and appreciation for the dentist and their team not only sets a good example but also helps in building a positive relationship between your family and the dental care providers.

Being kind and encouraging during your child's dental appointment is essential. Your supportive presence, combined with respectful and calm communication, can create a reassuring environment for your child. This approach not only helps in making the current visit more pleasant but also plays a vital role in shaping your child's attitude towards dental care in the future.

Careful with Your Words: Choosing Language Wisely

The language you use during your child's dental appointment can have a significant impact on their comfort and anxiety levels. Especially when it comes to potentially frightening aspects of dental care, like injections or 'shots', it's crucial to be mindful of your words. Here's how to navigate your language to keep the experience positive.

Avoid Mentioning 'Shots' or Other Scary Terms

Bringing up 'shots,' 'needles,' or any other terms associated with pain or discomfort can instantly create fear and anxiety in your child. Most dentists are skilled in using non-threatening language to explain these procedures to children. They often use child-friendly terms and metaphors that make the experience seem less intimidating. For example, a shot may be referred to as a 'sleepy juice' that helps the tooth nap while the dentist works.

Trust the Dentist's Communication

Allow the dentist to lead the conversation when it comes to explaining procedures to your child. They are trained to communicate in a way that is understandable and non-frightening to a child. Observe the language they use and support this by repeating or rephrasing it in your conversations with your child. This consistency in language between you and the dental team can help maintain a calm and reassuring environment.

Reinforce Positive Aspects

Focus your language on the positive aspects of the visit. Talk about how clean and healthy their teeth will be after the visit, or how the dentist is helping to keep their smile bright. Encourage them by praising their bravery and cooperation.

Prepare for Questions

If your child asks about something that could be scary, like shots or drills, frame your response in a reassuring and simple way. For example, you might say that the dentist has special tools to make sure their teeth are strong and healthy, and they always make sure the child is comfortable.

Model Calm and Positive Language

Children often mirror the behavior and language of their parents. By using calm and positive language yourself, you set an example for your child. This approach shows them that there's nothing to be afraid of and that they can trust the dental team.

The words you choose during your child's dental visit matter. By avoiding mentions of scary or painful procedures and supporting the dentist's child-friendly communication, you help create a more positive and less intimidating experience. This careful choice of language not only helps in reducing your child's dental anxiety but also builds their confidence in dental visits.

Respect Office Policy: Supporting Your Child's Independence

Dental offices, especially those specializing in pediatric dentistry, often have specific policies in place for the well-being of their young patients. One such policy might be that parents are not allowed in the treatment area, or operatory, during the appointment. While this might initially seem daunting, it's important to respect and support these guidelines for the benefit of your child. If this is something that you will just not be comfortable with make sure you ask about it beforehand.

Understanding the Policy

Firstly, understand the rationale behind such a policy. Dentists have observed that many children tend to behave better and are more cooperative when they are on their own. This behavior could be due to the children trying to assert independence or because they're less distracted without their parents. The dental team is trained to provide a supportive and safe environment for your child, focusing entirely on their care and comfort.

Preparing Your Child

If you're aware that the dental office has this policy, prepare your child beforehand. Talk to them about what will happen and assure them that the dentist and their team are friendly and professional. Emphasize how brave they are for going in alone and that you're just outside waiting for them.

Offer Reassurance

Before they go in, reassure your child of your presence. Let them know you'll be right there waiting for them once they're done. This reassurance can provide them with the confidence they need to face the situation independently.

Be Supportive and Positive

Show your support by being positive about the experience. Tell your child how proud you are of them for being so brave and independent. Your confidence in their ability to handle the situation will boost their self-esteem.

Respect and Trust the Dental Team

It's important to trust and respect the expertise of the dental team. They have experience in handling various situations with children and are skilled in making the dental visit a positive experience. If you have any concerns, discuss them with the dentist beforehand, but once the appointment starts, try to put your trust in their professional judgment.

Stay Calm

Even if you feel anxious about not being with your child, try to remain calm and composed. Your child will likely sense your emotions, and seeing you calm can help them feel more relaxed about the situation.

Respecting the dental office's policy about parents staying out of the operatory can be an opportunity for your child to demonstrate their bravery and independence. By preparing them for what to expect, offering reassurance, and showing your trust in the dental team, you help create a positive and empowering experience for your child. This approach not only supports the smooth running of the dental appointment but also contributes to your child's overall confidence and self-reliance.

Respond Positively to Dental Findings: Handling Cavities with Care

Discovering that your child has a cavity or two can be a concern, but the way you respond to these findings is crucial. It's important to handle such situations without inducing shame or fear in your child. Your response should be constructive and supportive, focusing on solutions rather than blame. Here's how to positively handle the news of cavities.

Avoid Expressing Disappointment or Blame

If the dentist informs you of a cavity, refrain from showing disappointment or frustration, both in your facial expressions and words. Avoid making statements that could make your child feel guilty or ashamed. Remember, cavities can happen despite good oral hygiene practices, and they are a common issue that can be addressed effectively.

Focus on Solutions

Shift the focus from the problem to the solution. Discuss with the dentist the steps to be taken to treat the cavity and ask about preventive measures for the future. Involve your child in this conversation in a child-friendly manner, emphasizing the positive aspect of fixing the problem and keeping their teeth healthy.

Reinforce Good Oral Hygiene Habits

Use this opportunity to gently reinforce the importance of good oral hygiene habits. Talk about brushing, flossing, and healthy eating in a positive light, making it a part of a routine for strong, healthy teeth. Frame it as a team effort, where you and your child work together to keep their teeth in great shape.

Offer Reassurance and Support

Let your child know that having a cavity is not the end of the world and that the dentist will take care of it. Reassure them that everyone gets cavities and it's just a sign that some extra care is needed for their teeth. Your support and reassurance can alleviate any fears or concerns they may have.

Educate Without Intimidation

Educate your child about cavities in a non-threatening way. You can explain that a cavity is a small spot on the tooth that needs to be cleaned and filled by the dentist so that their tooth can be strong again. Avoid using language that might scare them, such as 'drilling' or 'pain.'

Praise Their Cooperation

Regardless of the dental findings, praise your child for their behavior and cooperation during the visit. This positive reinforcement is important for building their confidence and making them feel good about their dental visits.

How you respond to the discovery of cavities is key to ensuring your child doesn't develop a negative association with dental visits. By focusing on solutions, reinforcing good habits, offering reassurance, and educating in a friendly manner, you can turn the situation into a constructive learning experience. Your supportive and positive approach will help your child maintain a healthy relationship with dental care.

In summary, your role during the dental appointment is to be a source of calm, encouragement, and support. By arriving early, maintaining a positive demeanor, avoiding fear-inducing topics, respecting the office's policies, and responding constructively to dental findings, you help create a positive experience for your child. This approach not only helps in making the current visit successful but also lays the groundwork for stress-free future appointments.

4

After The Appointment

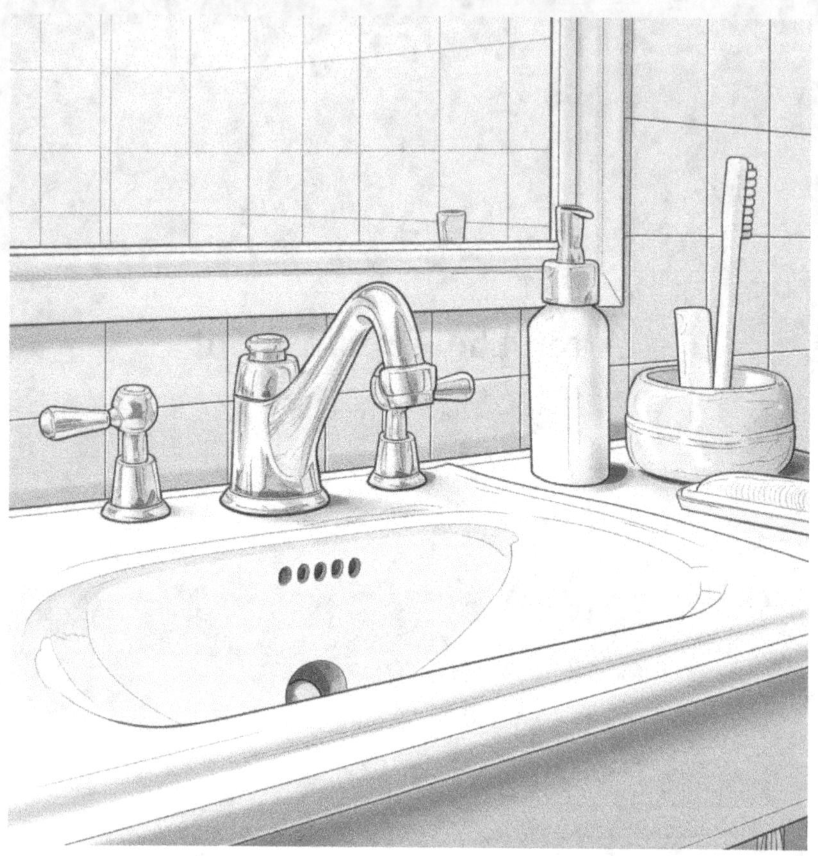

The dental appointment might be over, but your role as a parent in supporting your child's dental health continues. Post-appointment, it's essential to reinforce the positive aspects of the visit, address any treatments that may be needed, and prepare your child for future dental care. This chapter focuses on how you can help your child apply what they've learned and maintain good oral health practices.

Avoid Shaming: Handling Treatment Needs with Sensitivity

Discovering that your child requires further dental treatment can be a source of concern for any parent. However, it's essential to approach this topic with your child in a manner that is free from shame or blame. How you discuss post-treatment needs can significantly influence your child's attitude towards dental care and their self-esteem.

Focus on Health, Not Blame

When discussing the need for further treatment, keep the conversation focused on health and well-being, rather than what went wrong. Avoid phrases that imply fault, like "If only you had brushed better, this wouldn't have happened." Instead, use language that emphasizes the positive action going forward, such as, "The dentist is going to help your teeth get even stronger."

Explain Treatments in a Positive Light

Take the time to explain why the treatment is necessary in a way that's easy for your child to understand. Frame it as a positive step towards maintaining a healthy mouth. For instance, if a cavity needs filling, you might say, "The dentist is going to clean a small spot on your tooth and fill it with a special material to keep it strong."

Reassure Your Child

Children might feel scared or upset about the need for further treatment. Offer reassurance that the dentist is there to help them and that everything will be done to ensure their comfort. Remind them of any positive experiences they've had at the dentist's office and how brave they've been.

Involve Your Child in the Process

Make your child a part of the process by allowing them to ask questions and express their feelings. This involvement can help demystify the treatment and give them a sense of control over the situation.

Set a Positive Example

Your response to the treatment plan sets the tone for your child's reaction. Approach it with a calm and positive attitude, showing that while dental treatments are sometimes necessary, they're not something to fear.

Encourage and Praise

Regardless of the treatment needed, continue to encourage good oral hygiene habits and praise your child for their efforts. Recognize the steps they're taking to improve their dental health, reinforcing that these treatments are just one part of taking care of their teeth.

Avoiding shaming in post-treatment discussions involves focusing on positive health outcomes, explaining treatments in a child-friendly manner, offering reassurance, involving your child in the conversation, setting a positive example, and continuing to encourage and praise good oral hygiene habits. This approach ensures that your child views dental treatments as a normal and manageable aspect of oral health care, free from fear or stigma.

Schedule Prompt Treatment: Demonstrating the Importance of Dental Health

Once your child's dentist has recommended further treatment, whether it's a filling, a sealant, or any other procedure, it's important to schedule it as soon as possible. Promptly arranging for these treatments not only addresses dental issues effectively but also sends a clear message to your child about the importance of dental health.

Showcase the Priority of Dental Health

By scheduling the recommended treatment without delay, you demonstrate to your child that their dental health is a top priority. It underscores the idea that taking care of one's teeth is not something to be postponed or taken lightly. This lesson in prioritization will help instill a sense of importance regarding their oral health that can last a lifetime.

Reduce Anxiety with Prompt Action

The longer you wait to schedule a treatment, the more time there is for anxiety to build up in your child's mind. Addressing dental issues promptly can help reduce any worries or fears your child might have about the procedure. It shows them that dental issues are manageable and nothing to be overly concerned about.

Prevent Dental Issues from Worsening

Delaying dental treatment can lead to worsening conditions, more complex procedures, and potentially more discomfort for your child. Scheduling promptly ensures that any dental issues are dealt with before they become more serious, reinforcing the idea of preventive care.

Maintain a Routine

Keeping a regular schedule with dental appointments, including follow-up treatments, helps establish and maintain a routine. This regularity can help demystify dental visits and treatments, making them a normal part of your child's health care routine.

Involve Your Child in the Process

When scheduling the treatment, consider involving your child in the process. Let them know when the appointment is and what to expect. This involvement can give them a sense of control and participation in their own health care.

Positive Framing of the Treatment

Frame the upcoming treatment in a positive light. For example, if your child needs a filling, you might say, "The dentist is going to fix a small part of your tooth so it's strong again. Isn't it great that we have dentists to do this?"

Scheduling prompt treatment for your child's dental needs is crucial. It demonstrates the importance of dental health, reduces anxiety, prevents worsening of dental issues, maintains a routine, involves your child in their own health care, and helps frame dental care in a positive light. By doing so, you're not just taking care of their immediate dental needs; you're also helping them develop a responsible and proactive attitude towards their health.

Reinforce Home Care: Implementing Dentist's Recommendations

After a dental appointment, an essential part of maintaining your child's oral health is reinforcing home care and following any special instructions given by the dentist. This reinforcement helps in solidifying good dental habits and ensures that your child's teeth remain healthy between visits. Here's how to effectively reinforce home care based on the dentist's guidance.

Review and Implement Dentist's Instructions

Start by reviewing the instructions and recommendations given by the dentist. These may include specific brushing or flossing techniques, dietary suggestions, or special treatments like fluoride rinses. Ensure you understand these instructions clearly—if you have any doubts, don't hesitate to contact the dental office for clarification.

Make Oral Hygiene a Fun Routine

Incorporate the dentist's recommendations into your child's daily routine in a way that is enjoyable. For example, when they brush for two minutes, use a fun timer or play a short song they like to time it. When they are flossing, try using flossers designed for kids, which can be easier and more fun to use.

Lead by Example

Children often mimic their parents' behaviors. Show them that you take your oral health seriously by practicing good dental hygiene yourself. Brush and floss with your child, making it a family activity. This not only teaches them the importance of regular dental care but also makes it a normal part of daily life.

Positive Reinforcement

Praise your child for following through with their dental care routine. Positive reinforcement can go a long way in encouraging them to continue these practices. You can create a reward system for consistent dental care, like a sticker chart, to motivate them further.

Educational and Engaging Activities

Use books, apps, or videos that educate about dental health in a fun and engaging way. These resources can reinforce what the dentist said and make learning about oral health more appealing to your child.

Regular Reminders and Check-ins

Regularly remind your child about the importance of following the dentist's instructions. Make it a part of everyday conversation. Also, periodically check in to see how they are doing with their new habits, offering help and encouragement as needed.

Address Challenges Patiently

If your child faces challenges in adapting to new dental routines, be patient. Change can take time. Address any struggles with understanding and support, and try different approaches if necessary to find what works best for them.

Reinforcing home care and following the dentist's special instructions are crucial in maintaining your child's oral health. By making dental care a fun and regular part of their routine, leading by example, offering positive reinforcement, using educational tools, providing regular reminders, and being patient with challenges, you help your child develop and maintain good dental habits that will benefit them for a lifetime.

Preparing for the Next Appointment: Building Positive Anticipation

Whether your child's next dental visit is for a scheduled treatment or a routine exam, preparing them in advance is key to ensuring a positive experience. Building anticipation and understanding for the next appointment helps alleviate any anxiety and sets the stage for a successful visit. Here's how to effectively prepare your child for their upcoming dental appointment.

Discuss the Purpose of the Next Visit

Begin by explaining the purpose of the next appointment in a positive and reassuring manner. If it's for treatment, such as a filling, frame it as a step towards keeping their teeth strong and healthy. For a routine exam, emphasize how these visits help the dentist ensure their teeth are growing just as they should.

Mark the Calendar

Involve your child in the process by marking the date on the calendar. This can help them mentally prepare for the visit and understand that it's an important event. You can even count down the days together as the appointment approaches.

Recall Positive Experiences

Remind your child of any positive aspects from their previous visits. Maybe they enjoyed a particular game in the waiting room, or perhaps they liked how their teeth felt after a cleaning. Focusing on these positive experiences can help build a sense of anticipation and ease any nerves.

Role-play the Upcoming Visit

Engage in role-playing activities to simulate the dental visit. You can pretend to be the dentist while your child plays the patient, or vice versa. This exercise not only makes the idea of going to the dentist more familiar but can also be a fun way to learn and practice dental care.

Review What to Expect

Go over what typically happens during a dental visit, using simple and positive language. Explain the steps in an age-appropriate way, and reassure them that you'll be there with them, or waiting close by, depending on the office policy.

Emphasize the Importance of Oral Health

Use this opportunity to discuss the importance of maintaining good oral health and how regular dental visits contribute to this. Reinforce the idea that the dentist is a friend who helps keep their teeth healthy.

Address Any Concerns or Fears

If your child expresses any concerns or fears about the upcoming visit, listen to them attentively and provide reassurance. Answer their questions honestly and calmly, reassuring them that the dental team will do everything to make them comfortable.

Plan a Reward or Fun Activity Afterwards

Consider planning a small reward or a fun activity for after the appointment. This gives your child something positive to look forward to and can serve as a motivation for getting through the visit.

Preparing your child for the next dental appointment involves discussing the purpose of the visit, marking the calendar, recalling positive experiences, role-playing, reviewing what to expect, emphasizing the importance of oral health, addressing concerns, and planning a post-visit reward or activity. By taking these steps, you help build a positive mindset around dental visits, easing any apprehensions and setting the foundation for successful future appointments.

In summary, the period after the dental appointment is crucial for reinforcing the positive aspects of dental care, addressing any necessary treatments, and preparing your child for future visits. By discussing treatments in a non-shaming way, scheduling prompt follow-ups, reinforcing home care practices, and setting a positive tone for future appointments, you're helping your child develop healthy oral habits and a positive attitude towards dental care. This post-appointment care is key to ensuring your child values and maintains good oral health.

5

Conclusion

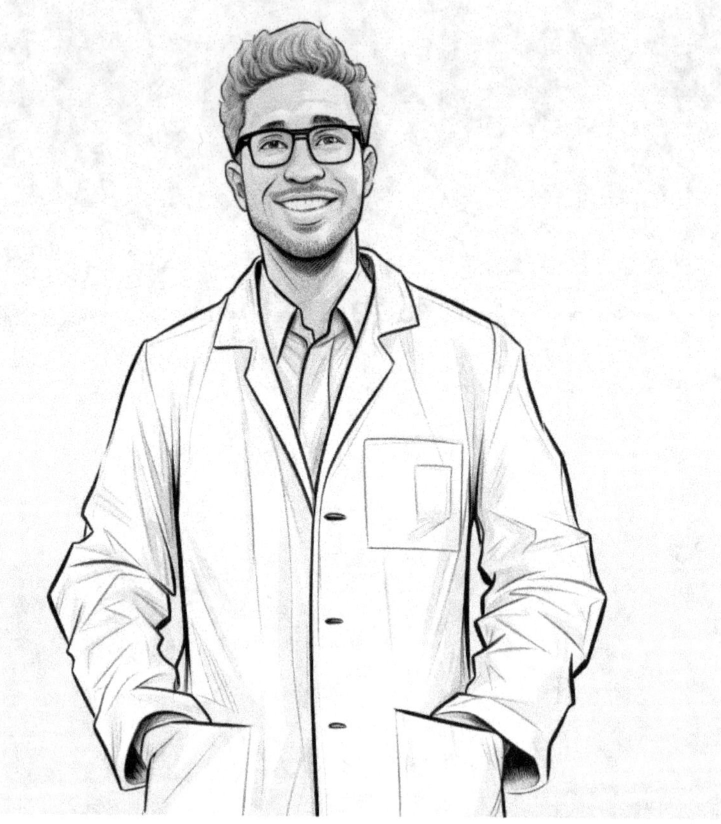

As we come to the end of this guide, it's my hope that this book has equipped you with valuable insights and practical strategies to transform dental visits from a source of anxiety into an opportunity for growth and learning for both you and your child.

From preparing for the first appointment to reinforcing positive dental habits at home, we've covered a range of topics aimed at demystifying the dental experience for your child. Remember, your role as a parent in this journey is pivotal. Your attitude, preparation, and the way you handle each step of the dental visit significantly influence your child's perception of dental care. By adopting the practices outlined in this guide, you are setting your child up for a lifetime of healthy teeth and positive dental experiences.

As you continue to apply these strategies, keep in mind that every child is unique, and what works for one may not work for another. Be patient, stay positive, and be willing to adapt as you learn what best suits your child's individual needs.

I encourage you to view dental care as an important part of your child's overall health and well-being. Regular dental visits, combined with good oral hygiene at home, are key to maintaining your child's dental health. And as they grow, the confidence and comfort they develop in the dentist's chair will serve them well into adulthood.

If you found this book helpful, please consider leaving a review on Amazon. Your feedback not only supports me as an author but also helps other parents find and benefit from these strategies. Sharing your experience can make a significant difference in another family's dental journey.

Thank you for joining me on this journey to making dental visits a positive experience for your child. Here's to many happy, healthy smiles in your family's future!

Sources

American Academy of Pediatric Dentistry. Policy on the dental home. The Reference Manual of Pediatric Dentistry. Chicago, Ill.: American Academy of Pediatric Dentistry; 2023:35-7.

Eye for Ebony. (n.d.). Girl wearing black vest raising two hands near green grass field during daytime [Photograph]. Unsplash. https://unspl ash.com/photos/girl-wearing-black-vest-raising-two-hands-near-gr een-grass-field-during-daytime-OWi1sIWiCAI utm_content=credit-ShareLink&utm_medium=referral&utm_source=unsplash

OpenAI. (2024). ChatGPT (GPT-4) [Software]. OpenAI. https://www.o penai.com/

Oral health policies and recommendations. (n.d.). https://www.aapd.o rg/research/oral-health-policies—recommendations/

Pexels. (n.d.). Kids smiling [Photograph]. Retrieved [01/17/2024], from https://www.pexels.com/search/kids%20smiling/